1

HEALING POWER OF COCONUT OIL

TABLE OF CONTENT

SUMMARY

CHAPTER-9   Pg.34

FREQUENTLY ASKED QUESTIONS.

Coco is a Spanish word that means monkey face. Resemblance of coconut with its three indentations and hairy nut to monkey's face; it started to be known as coconut. Coconut has innumerable health benefits and uses. Due to coconut's long and much respected history, around 1 / 3 of human population around the world depend to a great extent in one way or the other on its supplies and production. 'The tree of life' was the name given to it by the Pacific Islanders and historically it was considered to have a cure for all diseases. Recent studies on this have revealed many hidden secrets for its healing powers. For thousands of years it has been used to treat many illnesses and diseases besides being used as a component of food.

It has proved not only to cure diseases but helpful in preventing many diseases. Other than these, coconut oil has been proved to be beneficial in different industrial uses due to its high gelling temperature and viscosity. Its long shelf life due to high resistance to rancidity makes it easier to store it for long period of time. To improve shelf life hydrogen molecule is added through a process called hydrogenation. This process increases the saturation of unsaturated fatty acids i. e. mono unsaturated and polyunsaturated fatty acids. Partial hydrogenation of these leads to synthesis of trans-fatty acids. Trans-fatty acids are responsible for causing cardiovascular diseases and conditions leading to it.

Therefore, coconut oil in its original natural condition is not at all bad for the heart but artificial and synthetic processing of it leads to making hydrogenated coconut oil saturated enough to have any kind of negative effects on dietary intakes leading to health problems. Virgin coconut oil and extra virgin coconut oil are free from trans-fats. These oils needed to be incorporated in all kinds of meal planning, beauty products, massaging and medicinal properties for their innumerable benefits and powerful natural effects.

It has been noted that people of Sri Lanka who consume high amounts of coconut and coconut products have one of the lowest heart disease rates. Due to this blaming coconut as the cause of heart disease is absolutely wrong and baseless when the main culprit is hydrogenation and saturation processes just to improve the flavors and increase its shelf life and consequently gaining more financial benefits. Scientific name for coconut is cocos nucifera. Coconut is slightly sweet in flavor and a dry kernel contains around 60 %- 65 % fats.

CHAPTER-1

Why Coconut – What Is It?

Coconut oil and components of coconut oil have typical distinguishing factors making them altogether highly valued due to these. Coconut oil has been used for centuries for its unique properties in many parts of the world and the wisdom of the wise kept on passing the goodness sealed within from one generation to the next. Due to its true medicinal value, a tree of coconut is considered a symbol of life and is a great source of coconut meat, milk, juice and oil. Coconut juice is a purest of all juices and sealed with perfection to furnish all the goodness inside. Its goodness has not been felt only inside the body but outer application through massage and in beauty products have been proved.

In medicine its component in the form of medium chain triglycerides commonly known as MCT oil has proven record that no other oil can compete. MCT oil can be added to naso-gastric feeds commonly known as NG feeds. It has many proven uses in industries as well where other types of fats failed to achieve the same results and this is only due to its unique composition which makes it different from the rest. It also possesses one more distinguishing quality among plant sources of fats and oils of having longest shelf life. It lasts longer than other oils and does not get rancid easily.

It has achieved a status of being a source of food and medicine among the people from all around the world speaking different languages, having different cultures, belonging to different religions and adhering to various traditions. Its beneficial uses have been traditionally passed on from one generation to another. 1 tbsp. Of coconut oil furnishes around 117 calories while 1 tbsp. of other oils furnishes around 135 calories. Therefore it is the only known fat that has lower caloric value as compared to either butter or any other hydrogenated vegetable oil source.

Coconut oil contains 92 % saturated fat. Pure virgin coconut oil can be solid, semi-solid or liquid depending upon the room temperature. It is made up of various fatty acids and contains lauric acid, myristic acid and capric acid. It may contain other beneficial chemical sources of plants that may get discovered through studies.

Only recently it has been studied in the light of science and scientific facts. Its real goodness has been rediscovered through scientific investigations and procedures. This ongoing process has been helpful in distinguishing between myths and facts. Scientific understanding knew that there is some truth behind the words of the wise based on centuries. Many researchers due to this dedicated their time, money and efforts to unfold the hidden truth. Many studies have been conducted in the area but still many more are needed to fully understand its potential for being unique in its own sense.

Presence of lauric acid in coconut oil in abundance makes it anti-bacterial, anti-viral, anti-fungal and anti-protozoal. Coconut fat contains around 50 % lauric acid which is a medium chain fatty acid. Monolaurin is being produced from lauric acid inside a human body which acts like anti-bacterial, anti-viral and anti-protozoal. Monoglycerides of lauric acid have shown even better results and are more effective than the fatty acid itself. Good thing about mono-laurine is that it does not destroy the gut bacteria which are desirable but only attacks the pathogenic micro-organisms.

Coconut fat contains about 6-7 % capric acid which is another kind of medium chain fatty acids. Inside a human body it is formed into mono-caprin which has shown to have antiviral effects against HIV. Capric acid has also been found to possess qualities of anti-microbial.

Coconut oil is one of the few natural plant sources of saturated fat and the kind of fat it possess is helpful in reducing the bad type cholesterol and increasing the good type cholesterol naturally. Types of fatty acids found in coconut oil have been recognized to have specific natural health renewal system that needs in-depth study and understanding. Some of the naturally occurring saturates found in coconut oil are found to be more beneficial than some of the unsaturated from other sources.

This leads to a conclusion that how could nature be challenged by labeling foods to be either good or bad. Therefore, all foods are good if eaten in balance and given due consideration to wide variety. Each food contains some kind of goodness missing from the others. Extremism in food intake and liking and disliking leads to deficiencies or over nourishment leading to obesity and consequently to many diseases.

Using coconut and its oil as wholesome or utilizing its various beneficial components e. g. lauric acid, capric acid or MCT , all have proved to be beneficial in one way or the other for many conditions and eliminating or reducing the effects of many diseases. It helps in soothing sore throat, works as a lip balm and provides relief from ear infection.

Virgin coconut oil has been found to provide protection to liver from various effects of drugs. . It has also been found to be beneficial in either eliminating or reducing problems associated with many chronic diseases and helping in providing alternative natural therapies without any due side effects. Many diseases and conditions in which it has been tried and tested and found to be of great benefits include GERD, chronic sinusitis, heart problems, Alzheimer, hemorrhoid, cancer, diabetes, psoriasis, gall bladder diseases, bladder infection, flu, athletic foot, ring worm, arthritis, Parkinson, etc. Each individual is unique and therefore each one's response to coconut therapy may be different and we also cannot expect coconut to be the cure for all diseases but one thing is certain that it is only a part of a diet and do not carry any type of side effects with it.

Coconut oil has also been found to be helpful in increasing the absorption of minerals and vitamins and other nutrients from the gut e. g. calcium, magnesium, fat soluble vitamins A, D, E, K, beta-carotene and few amino acids. In this way it is indirectly responsible for reducing undernourishment and deficiencies.

Coconut oil can be consumed through dietary intake. Adding it in many dishes can create great recipes. It can also be consumed directly through tea spoon full or table spoon full once or twice daily respectively. Its daily intake is important for good health, protection from infection and to avoid many health problems, conditions and diseases.

It has also been found to prevent stretch marks of pregnancy, support thyroid function and provide relief from psoriasis, eczema, varicose veins, depression, autism, allergy symptoms, cellulites, anxiety, baby rash, sleep disorders, decreased mental alertness, etc.

Coconut oil has high smoking point and it also possesses anti insect repellent properties. It improves memory, regulates hormones, reduces wrinkles, heals wounds, reduces epileptic seizures, dissolves kidney stones, improves digestion, etc.

A coconut palm is from a family of Arecaceae and in the genus cocos it is the only accepted specie. It is commonly found in the tropical and subtropical areas. Due to its versatility of various uses of its different parts, it is well known for its high value.

Coconut is being consumed in many parts of the world as staple food. Coconut fruit contains large amount of water when mature and are different from other fruits. Immature coconut fruit contains tender nuts and could be consumed as a drink. The hard outside shell can be used as charcoal. The dried coconut flesh is called copra. Oil derived from the hard nut can be used for cooking, frying and baking. Coconut milk and cream can also be used in a variety of ways in cookery.

Coconut oil is also used in a variety of ways in the manufacture of soaps and cosmetics. Coconut water, a clear liquid is a refreshing drink. The leaves, husks, shell and its wood is used to manufacture many goods and products. Countries which are great suppliers of coconut and its products include Philippines, Malaysia, Indonesia, India, Maldives, Polynesia, and southern Asia. It is also commonly found in South America, Pacific Island, Hawaii and Florida.

All parts of a coconut tree is beneficial in one way or the other and therefore its tree is supposed to supply everything needed for a living. Coconut fruit has a variety of food uses e. g. coconut meat, cream, milk, sugar, water and oil. The shell is also utilized as a bowl, dish or cup. The fibers of seeds are used in the making of brushes, mats, fishnets and rope.

It takes around one whole year for a coconut to mature but the tree blooms thirteen times per year. Coconuts are continuously formed and harvest is available the year round. An average harvest from one tree is 60 coconuts and many trees yield three times this amount. It is considered to be a drupe and not a nut. Some coconut trees are tall and some are dwarfs. Fruits from dwarfs are eaten fresh while fruits from tall trees are used for the supply of coconut oil and fiber.

The dwarf trees tend to account for only 5 percent of coconut. They are self-fertilizing, produce rounded sweet fruit, are being self-pollinated and have domesticated traits. It is difficult to track the origins of cultivation due to the long history of human interaction with coconuts.

CHAPTER-2

Common Coconut Oil Myths

Many common coconut oil myths are attached to it due to miss-understandings and many due to artificial hype created by vested interest groups for various economy factors related to it. Whatever the reasons behind one thing is certain that due to this many have been deprived of its so many blessings showered upon humanity by nature's gift and will keep on depriving if kept in darkness. One more reason leading towards this is by artificial saturation process of hydrogenation leading to reduced beneficial effects and increased harmful effects which could easily be avoided. But this has been the most neglected issue not only towards coconut oil but all sorts of vegetable oils. Strict policy development on universal basis and adherence to it is urgently required by the policy makers to avoid further damage occurring due to this.

Hydrogenation process is the culprit behind synthetic saturation of oils leading to production of trans- fatty acids. Trans-fatty acids have proven record of causing all sorts of diseases. No one would like to compromise on health just for the sake of the flavor of the food. There are thousands of ways to improve the flavor without compromising on health. Besides improving the flavor, hydrogenation process is also responsible to increase the viscosity and shelf life. Increased viscosity also leads to increased market acceptability and majority of the public being ignorant finds these more appealing. Many people start blaming the oil instead of the processing behind. For this, more awareness programs are needed in all the nook and corner of the world.

Only to make these oils more marketable and gain more profits these kinds of processes and tactics are applied without giving due consideration to its harmful effects on humanity. This is happening throughout the world and no particular area can be blamed but each one is effected even after knowing. The process of hydrogenation of oils needed to be banned if we want the chances of decreased obesity, hypertension, cardiovascular and many other diseases to increase. Many food authorities have taken measurable actions against it and many are requiring proper labeling of the content of foods to decrease incidences of these diseases.

There is no credible scientific support available against coconut or coconut oil causing any kind of negative effects. It is untrue to suggest coconut does not possess healing powers when it has been time and again proven record through research studies showing it to have natural antibiotic and anti-oxidative properties. Just black listing it due to its natural saturation properties is not enough to label it heart enemy oil.

One myth involving coconut oil and its consumption is associated with weight gain and it is believed mistakenly that it helps in weight gain and obesity which is not at all true. Medium chain fatty acids present in coconut oil helps in increasing the metabolic rate and energy is being consumed at a higher level and more energy is spent and released and more fat is being utilized.

Coconut oil does not raise the bad type cholesterol and protects the heart towards developing atherosclerosis or developing conditions leading to heart diseases.

Many people also believe that coconut oil irritates skin which is not at all true. It actually protects the skin from all kinds of itching and irritation. It helps in soothing the skin in case of inflammation caused by insect bites, sun burn, allergies, bruises and reaction of drugs. The anti-microbial properties associated with coconut oil helps in healing wounds and fight off infection.

One more myth attached with coconut oil is that it is sweet and cannot be consumed by diabetics. Coconut oil does not contain glucose and is not at all sweet. In fact this oil promotes secretion of insulin from the pancreas and reduces the chances to develop diabetes greatly.

Many people also believe that coconut oil is thick in cold climatic conditions and do not get easily absorbed by the skin. In fact this is totally untrue as it becomes liquid as it comes into contact with the skin temperature and gets readily absorbed by the skin and is preferred for massaging and tanning.

Many myths are also associated with its shelf life. As it is obtained from coconut which is high in moisture content it has short shelf life and gets rancid easily. This is untrue and coconut oil has long shelf life and do not get rancid easily. In fact it has the longest shelf life amongst most of the oils from plant origins. If unopened it may last for three to four years and opened bottle can last for at least two years. If refrigerated and unopened can even last for eight to ten years without getting rancid.

One more myth associated with this oil is that it tastes bad. Most of the people who have tasted it believe that it tastes very good. One can fry a thing in coconut oil and try out and will understand how good it tastes.

CHAPTER-3

Health Benefits of Coconut Oil

Coconut oil has been able to recover from blameworthy situation of being heart enemy to heart friendly. Just because it was naturally saturated it was thought that it might have negative effects on our heart which was proved to be totally wrong after various studies and researches found out the truth. The kind of saturated fat it is and many of its constituents helps in decreasing many kinds of diseases mainly cardiac and obesity.

Heart diseases

The presence of lauric acid in coconut oil helps in increasing the serum HDL level which is good type cholesterol. Numerous health benefits of coconut and its oil and derivatives of its oils are well known through population studies especially its role in decreasing heart diseases and increasing resistance to many diseases. It has some inbuilt chemical power that makes it differ from the rest and most probably its unique fatty acid composition makes it hard to ignore for its all beneficial medicinal properties known from centuries. Many studies have proved it to be beneficial in many conditions but many still are under way.

Coconut oil has also been seen to have a cholesterol lowering action by converting it to pregenolone. Pregenalone is a molecule which is a precursor for many hormones that a human body needs. Most of the therapeutic value of coconut lies in its fat content.

Abnormal thyroid function can be a cause for increase in bad type cholesterol. Coconut oil helps in normalizing and regulating the thyroid function. It also helps in reducing stress and sore throat.

Coconut oil has also been associated with having an effect of lowering the amount of belly fat. Abdominal fat stores are associated with cardiovascular problems and this fat is even difficult to lose.

Although 92 % of naturally occurring coconut oil is saturated fat, but it has been found to provide protection against heart attacks and strokes. It has also been associated with giving strength to bones.

Non hydrogenated naturally occurring coconut oil helps in improving the cholesterol profile of blood.

According to various researches based on population studies people who have been traditionally consuming large amounts of coconut and coconut oil have low to very low incidences of cardiovascular diseases and their serum cholesterol level remain within normal ranges.

Studies have also revealed the presence of Medium Chain Fatty Acids MCFA in coconut oil for being responsible for protection against heart diseases.

Many studies have also revealed that coconut consumption has been resulting in lowering heart diseases, improving cholesterol levels, lowering fat deposits, increasing rate of survival, reducing blood clot tendency, lessening uncontrolled free radicals in cell, improving anti-oxidant reserves, decreasing incidences of cardiovascular diseases, etc.

Atherosclerosis or hardening of arteries due to the presence of plaque can be a cause leading towards heart attacks. One of the causes of atherosclerosis is chronic bacterial and viral infection. As antibiotics are only effective towards bacteria and not viruses it has limited potential to deal with the situation. On the other hand coconut and coconut products have been found to be effective against not only bacteria but viruses as well as other microbes. It works to fight against these pathogens causing chronic infections. Regular intake of coconut and its derivatives and products have a role to play in one way or the other to revert any kind of chronic infections leading to atherosclerosis and consequently towards coronary artery diseases.

Many population studies have resulted in direct correlation between consumption of coconut oil and reduced rates of heart disease and consumption of other oils and fats with increased rates of heart diseases. Same population which had lower risks of heart disease due to high consumption of coconut, coconut oil and its products traditionally started showing signs of increased incidences of these diseases due to increased intake of other types of fats and oils.

Therefore we can conclusively say that increased intake of coconut and its products are directly associated with decreased levels of cardiovascular diseases. They provide hidden powers of protection that need to be understood and studied.

Weight Loss

Eating coconut and incorporation of coconut oil in many food items increases the basal metabolic rate. It has also been associated with reduced belly fat which correlates with decreased heart diseases. Fat and fatty acids of coconut oil get easily metabolized and are less likely to get stored in the body in the form of adipose tissues. Fatty acids of coconut oil prefer to get burnt for energy than getting stored. They are also helpful in reducing malnourished.

Stimulation of thermo-genesis by dietary intake of coconut oil in the form of MCT leads to weight loss due to increased energy expenditure. This has been proven through many studies. Increased intake of medium chain fatty triglycerides has been found to have an effect of increased energy expenditure and fat oxidation. According to scientific studies fatty acids from coconut oil are not easily converted to stored body fat but instead get readily utilized by the body.

Coconut oil is directly associated with increased basal metabolic rate leading towards weight loss as weight gain is directly associated with sluggish basal metabolic rate. The presence of lauric acid is invaluable. Lauric acid is also found in mother's milk.

Studies conducted have also revealed that coconut oil helps in reducing belly fat which is otherwise difficult to reduce and is beneficial in prevention and treatment of obesity and overweight.

CHAPTER-4

Coconut Oil For Healthy Skin And Hair.

Coconut oil helps in providing best nourishment needed for having healthy hair and skin. It keeps the renewal process at peak and provides protection from varying atmospheric conditions. It improves the luster of hair by giving them more shine and making them more soft, smooth and silky. It also acts like a natural conditioner and moisturizer that keep dandruff at bay.

Massaging your hair once or twice a week has been found to be helpful in relieving mental stress as well. The same good results have been reported for massaging this oil on face, ears and neck. Our head and face are directly related to our senses and mental capabilities. In addition to having great benefits through internal ingestion it is well qualified to possess hidden secrets of healing power through outer application. Coconut and coconut oil can be called a great natural gift to humanity.

Coconut oil improves skin texture, clears complexion and brightens radiance. It gets easily absorbed by the skin and removes any dryness and makes it soft and healthy. It is usually suitable for all kinds of complexion and skin types. Solidified coconut can be melted through hot water bath in cold climatic conditions as well as could be used in the solid form. The presence of fat soluble vitamins and its fatty acid combination have been tried and tested to provide natural source of nourishment to the skin and hair.

Massaging the head with coconut oil few hours before shampooing can have remarkable results. Even better results can be achieved by leaving it overnight for its soothing effects on brain. Precautionary measures needed to be taken if you want to avoid any kind of undesirable stains and spots on your pillows. You may protect it by covering it with an old shirt or towel.

When using coconut oil on your face you do not have to be careful about avoiding the eye area as it is a natural source and does not possess any kind of harmful effects on any part of the body. With artificial and synthetic creams and lotion one has to be careful as they contain chemicals and synthetic compounds.

CHAPTER-5

How Does Coconut Oil Work In Various Diseases?

Presence of lauric acid has been recognized to possess natural antibiotic properties and has been related to its anti-bacterial, antiviral and anti-protozoa properties. Coconut oil is a rich source of lauric acid. Usage of it in the diet has been associated with protection against alcohol damage and improving the immune system.

The presence of the combination of fatty acids in coconut helps it to support many health functions. The requirement made to label the products containing trans-fats will help in gaining better reputation for coconut and its products. Now coconut oil will be able to compete in a better manner and gain position that might help it to increased utilization by the baking and snacking industry. Coconut creams and desiccated coconut are 69 % coconut fat while coconut milk is around 24 % fat.

50 % of the fatty acids in coconut oil include lauric acid which is a medium chain fatty acid. Lauric acid can convert into mono-laurin inside the human body which is mono-glycerides which acts as antiviral, antibacterial and antiprotozoal. They have the capability of destroying the lipid coated viruses e. g. HIV, cytomegalovirus, influenza, herpes,

and many pathogenic bacteria including helicobacter pylori and protozoa such as giardia lamblia.

Coconut oil contains about 6-7 % of capric acid. Capric acid is a medium chain fatty acid having similar beneficial effects when converted to mono caprin inside the body. Mono-caprin also acts like antiviral against HIV and have antibacterial effects against many bacterial diseases.

The hype created against coconut due to its natural saturated properties has led many misunderstanding and myths. Due to this people have been deprived of many of its beneficial effects for a very long period of time. Compulsory labeling of products containing trans-fats will help coconut to regain its lost glory. Many consumers remained deprived of its natural properties and making best use of it in their daily lives.

Since nearly last four decades researchers have known the anti-viral, anti-bacterial and anti-protozoa properties of lauric acid and mono-laurin resulting in more than twenty research papers and numerous patents. A larger group of scientists, clinician and nutritionists have been largely unaware of the full potentials of coconut and coconut oil and many properties of providing diet therapy and various healing factors.

People have started to learn more about it recently. Mono-glycerides and derivatives of medium chain fatty acids can have adverse effects on many micro-organisms e. g. bacteria, fungi, yeast, viruses, etc. Structure of lipids helps in determining its anti-infective actions and mono-glycerides being active while triglycerides are inactive. Myristic acid and capric acid present in coconut oil have lower anti- virus actions than lauric acid which has greater anti-virus action. Lauric acid is saturated and found in abundance in coconut oil.

Fatty acids and mono-glycerides produce their inactivating and killing effect by lysing the plasma membrane. Mono-laurin solubilize the lipids and phospholipids in the envelope of viruses and disintegrates the viral envelop. The lipid membrane of the viruses is being disrupted by the action of medium chain saturated fatty acids and their derivatives. HIV, herpes virus, measles virus and vesicular stomatitis virus are some of the viruses that could be inactivated by these lipids.

These fatty acids and their derivatives are totally non-toxic to human due to being a natural substance. Lauric acid is one of the best inactivating fatty acids and its derivative mono-glycerides is even better. Mono-laurin does not affect the good type gut bacteria but only attacks the pathogenic ones. Mono-laurin has the capacity to inactivate many pathogenic bacteria including Listeria mono-cytogenes, Staphylococcus aureus, Streptococcus agalactiae, Streptococci- groups A, F, and G, some gram negative organisms and some gram positive organisms.

CHAPTER-6

Alternative Uses Of Coconut And Coconut Oil

Besides dietary and medicinal uses there are various other industrial uses of coconut, coconut oil and its derivatives. A coconut palm tree is supposed to carry more than thousand uses. An eye for innovation is still needed to look for many undiscovered hidden treasures in it. Due to its versatility it has been used for various purposes from building material to jet fuel. It is also being incorporated to produce many cosmetic items.

It has various industrial uses e. g. used in synthesis and production of creams, lotions, detergents, soaps, toothpaste, biofuel, lubricants, deodorants, shampoo, motor oil, bio diesel fuel, engine lubricant, lamp fuel, wood polish, conditioner for wood cutting board, rust inhibitor, bronze polish, plastic,   grease, resins, solvents, etc. It is also being used as natural after shave lotion.

It has also been used to power diesel as well as petrol engines as alternative oil and did not cause any problem to the engine. This alternative source of oil has also proved to be environment friendly.

Acid derivatives of coconut oil can also be used as natural herbicide.

Coconut oil is also being used as fuel to generate electricity.

It can be used as a cleanser to clean hands and brush after painting.

CHAPTER-7

Treatment Of Ailments

Coconut oil helps in the treatment of many common ailments like cold and flu by acting as a natural anti biotic. It is also known to cure many ailments efficiently due to its typical healing and health giving natural properties. It is a natural medicine with no side effects. It helps in providing sustenance with improved satiety and better metabolism.

It kills or expels lice, giardia, tapeworm and parasites. It provides quick bursts of energy, increases endurance and improves physical activity. It lessens problems associated with cystic fibrosis, etc. It also helps in preventing tooth decay and aids in immune system, prevents liver and kidney diseases, dissolves kidney stones, protects against bladder infection, provides protection against degenerative diseases and premature aging.

It is also beneficial in Alzheimer's disease in which the brain cells are unable to utilize the energy of glucose, therefore they need ketone bodies as an alternative source of energy to function properly. MCT oil a coconut derivative helps in furnishing constant amount of ketones without fasting or ketosis.

Gastro- Esophageal Reflux Disease commonly known as GERD is caused by Helico Pylori Bacteria inhibits the stomach and the esophagus and causes excessive production of hydrochloric acid or gastric juice. This can be painful and can lead to gastritis, ulcers and rarely gastric cancer. Coconut oil works as a natural antibiotic and kills the acid forming bacteria naturally. Fatty acids present in coconut oil kills H. Pylori due to being highly anti- bacterial.

It is also known to improve blood sugar level and risks associated with diabetes. Many symptoms associated with Crohn's disease can also be relieved. Reduces many symptoms associated with gall bladder disease, pancreatitis, hemorrhoids, etc.

CHAPTER-8

Summary

Coconut and many of coconut derivatives have numerous health and industrial uses. It being a natural source does not pose any kind of adverse health effects. It has much dietary and medicinal therapeutic value. In many food items it can be added in place of other sources of fats for its many beneficial effects and uses. I can also be consumed raw to boast energy and to provide protection against many infections and common ailments. Beside internal benefits it has been known for centuries to possess various outer application benefits.

It provides nourishment to the skin, hair and nails. It is a best type of replacement for artificial and synthetic lotions and cream. It does not possess any kind of synthetic compounds therefore do not possess any kind of health risks. It helps in providing protection against many disease causing germs and bacteria and helps to recover from many diseases by enhancing natural defense mechanism and improving immunity. It helps in increasing the basal metabolic rate and therefore is beneficial in reducing weight and prevention of obesity. It is excellent baby massage oil and can also be used to combat diaper rash.

Its various unusual properties lie in its fat content and the types of fatty acids it possess. Three main types of fatty acids found in coconut and its oil include lauric acid, capric acid and myristic acid. It is a natural saturated fat and therefore in cold climate gets solidified at room temperature. It has pleasant aroma and flavor. It does not get rancid easily and have long shelf life. It is mostly white in color with wax like texture.

For centuries people living around the world have known to benefit from it in one way or the other. The wood of the tree is also being used to construct houses. Its typical viscosity, melting point, smoking point and chemical content vary it from the rest. Every part of the tree is a blessing in its own sense and being utilized in one way or the other. It has also been tested positively as jet fuel.

According to many studies coconut and coconut oil does not lead to high serum cholesterol level. It is also not a cause for high coronary heart disease. Coconut oil can be used in a variety of ways in the cookery. Baking can be done using this oil instead of other types of fats and oils. It can also be used to pop popcorns and in the making of chocolates.

Coconut oil contains 91 % of saturated fatty acids, 6 % of mono unsaturated fatty acids and 3 % of polyunsaturated fatty acids. It has a smoking temperature of 35 degrees Fahrenheit.

Coconut oil and all derivatives or fractions of coconut oil are beneficial for one reason or the other. Medium chain triglycerides commonly known as MCT oil have many medical applications.

2.5 % of the total world plant oil production comes through coconut oil. Virgin coconut oil VCO is produced by not altering the oil obtained from mature fresh coconut kernel.

Serving size of coconut oil is 100gm which furnishes around 862 calories. It has been used successfully as a diesel engine fuel and can also supply fuel for electricity generation. Philippines is currently using coconut as a fuel for transportation. It has also been used as an engine lubricant. Acid derivatives of coconut oil can be used as a natural herbicide.

As a natural substance it has been known to extend youth. Coconut oil kills disease producing germs and helps in curing many skin, nail and hair problems. It supports the function of thyroid. It also helps in improving blood pressure. It gives strength to bones by helping in better calcium absorption, provides better diabetic control, and prevents cancer.

Coconut can either be eaten raw or can be incorporated into many dishes. It is biodegradable, is light in color and has pleasant flavor and aroma.

Coconut is especially beneficial for skin and many skin diseases. It makes it soft, gives radiance, shine and glow and protects it from heat and climatic conditions. It gets easily absorbed by the skin and helps in improving its color and texture.

It can also be used in oil lamps and the flame does not leave smoke. It is also used in the manufacture of soaps, liquid soaps, shampoo, shaving creams and many cosmetics. It does not contain cholesterol as it is a plant source and it contains vitamin E. It is also used in the manufacture of baby foods.

Coconut oil is made up of medium chain fatty acids or medium chain triglycerides and can easily be burnt to furnish energy. It is stable, is resistant to oxidation and contain low amount of polyunsaturated fatty acids when consumed along with its kernel helps in reducing total serum cholesterol.

It also helps in the absorption of vitamins, minerals and amino acids. Medium and short chain fatty acids containing less than 12 carbon atoms contribute to more than 70 % of the saturated fatty acids found in coconut oil.

Coconut oil is a natural saturated fat from plant which does not possess same risk factors as animal saturated fatty acids. Naturally occurring coconut oil do not possess trans-fatty acids.

It improves insulin efficiency, furnishes quick energy and do not get stored as adipose tissues easily. It also acts like anti parasitic effects, helps in digestion, improves bowel movement and regulates hormones. It also helps in building cells, provides protection from wrinkles and memory loss. Coconut oil helps in retaining youth for a longer period of time.

Coconut water is 100 % sterile and pure. It has highest concentration of naturally occurring electrolytes therefore it is an excellent source of re hydration. It helps the skin to get naturally get rid of the dangerous toxins and helps it to stay smooth, healthy and younger looking for a longer period of time.

It also provides protection against dental cavities and chewing one inch square piece of coconut meat on daily basis helps in keeping the teeth and gums strong.

Coconut oil contains high concentration of short chain and medium chain fatty acids which are necessary for good health. Due to coconuts high fiber content it can add good amount of fiber if added to a diet. It has low glycemic index and helps in maintaining blood glucose level. It reduces cravings for sweets and provides satiety for a longer period of time.

It is a quick source of energy, does not contain trans-fats, is gluten free, hypoallergenic, antibacterial, anti-viral, anti-fungal, and anti-parasitic and supports immune system, healing of wounds and speeds up recovery. It has natural property to work as anti-ulcer, anti-inflammatory, fever reducing and analgesic.

It also possesses brain boosting, fat burning and belly fat reducing property. Approximately one thousand mature coconuts weigh around 1440 kilograms and yield around 70 liter coconut oil and 370g coconut powder. In fractionated coconut oil, a fraction of the whole oil is separated for a variety of uses. Different medium chain fatty acids are separated e. g. lauric acid and capric acid. Lauric acid is a 12 carbon chain fatty acid and is separated for many industrial and medical uses. Capric acid is also fractionated for various different uses e. g. for different diets, medical use, cosmetics and fragrances.

The roots of coconut are beneficial for medicinal use. Its trunk is used to make houses, decorative items, furniture, etc. Coconut leaves can be used to produce high quality natural goods e. g. brooms, paper, hats, mats, fruit trays, hand fans, decorative items, lamp shades, bags, etc.

Flowers, seeds and roots of coconut are used to prepare creams, infusions and pastes for medicinal purposes. Fruit juice is mixed with rice flour and heated and is applied to gangrenous ulcers and skin boils. Fermented juice is being taken as a laxative. The roots are used as an infusion for sore throat gargles. Seeds of coconut are used to treat skin and nasal ulcers.

Coconut oil is applied to scalp to encourage new hair growth and to prevent premature graying. Coconut water mixed with olive oil can be used to get rid of intestinal parasites. It helps in soothing ear ache when mixed with garlic oil and olive oil. Coconut oil supports and repair tissues and reduces muscle and joint inflammation.

CHAPTER-9

Frequently Asked Questions

Q 1. Is coconut oil a saturated fat?

A 1. Yes, coconut oil is a saturated fat.

Q 2. Is it bad for heart?

A 2. Virgin coconut oil is not bad for the heart. Try to avoid all sorts of hydrogenated fats as they contain trans-fatty acids which can be harmful for the health of the heart.

Q 3. Is eating coconut, coconut cream and milk as beneficial as coconut oil?

A 3. Eating whole coconut is even more beneficial due to the presence of fiber and other content.

Q 4. Can I drink coconut oil as a supplement?

A 4. Yes, you can consume 1-2 tsp. of coconut oil twice or thrice a day.

Q 5. Can coconut oil protect me from various diseases?

A 5. Yes coconut oil has a unique quality of providing protection against various diseases. It works like a natural anti-biotic without having any side effects.

Q 6. Can it reduce weight?

A 6. Use it instead of other oils as it helps in increasing basal metabolic rate. Yes it will help in reducing weight especially belly fat.

Q 7. Can it be used as a skin moisturizer?

A 7. Yes it can be used as a skin moisturizer and especially good for dry flaky skin.

Q 8. Can it be used as oil for hair massage?

Q 8. It is excellent oil for hair massage. It helps in reducing mental stress and depression. It also helps in increasing mental alertness and reducing dandruff.

Q 9. Does it possess any kind of harmful effects?

A 9. It is a natural substance and therefore does not possess any kind of harmful effects.

Q 10. Can it be beneficial in the treatment of dandruff?

A 10. Yes it helps in the controlling and treatment of dandruff.

Q 11. Does it increase bad type cholesterol?

A 11. No it does not increase bad type cholesterol.

Q 12. Can it help in reducing seizure attacks?

A 12. Yes it is known to reduce seizure attacks.

Q 13. Can it work as a natural herbicide?

A 13. Yes it can work as a natural herbicide.

Q 14. Does coconut oil possess therapeutic value?

A 14. Yes it does possess therapeutic value.

Q 15. Can it be used as a diesel engine fuel?

A 15. Yes it can be used as a diesel engine fuel.